Diabetes & Hypertension Cookbook:

45 Recipes for Low Carb / Low Salt Diet

Annie DePasquale, MD

FREE BONUS

As a small token of appreciation for purchasing this book, Dr. Annie would like to offer you a free copy of her next health-related e-book.

You can get your free gift by clicking here:

http://www.FamilyDocAnnie.com/cookbook

© 2018 Annie DePasquale

All rights reserved. No portion of this book may be reproduced in any form without permission from the publisher, except as permitted by U.S. Copyright law.

For permissions contact: FamilyDocAnnie@gmail.com

Visit the author's website at http://www.FamilyDocAnnie.com

Disclaimer

The information in this book is for informational purposes only, and is not intended to serve as a substitute for the medical treatment of a qualified physician or healthcare provider.

Acknowledgements

This book is dedicated to my primary care patients who work so hard every single day to control their diabetes and blood pressure. You all are truly inspiring.

Introduction

Hi, I'm Annie DePasquale, a family medicine physician in Washington, D.C., who is extremely passionate about helping my patients who have diabetes and hypertension.

A few weeks ago, I looked on Amazon to see if there were any good books published about how to eat well if you have both diabetes and hypertension. I was surprised to find none. This motivated me to put together a cookbook that would be able to help people who are trying to keep a low carbohydrate and low salt diet.

I hope that you enjoy the recipes and that they help you to live a happy and healthier life.

Sincerely,

Dr. Annie

TABLE OF CONTENTS

BREAKFAST MEALS 9
   Oven- Baked Spinach and Tomato Omelet 9
   Turnip Breakfast a Notch 11
   Egg Puff French Toast Twist 13
   Breakfast Ball Sandwich 15
   Avocado Breakfast Burrito 17
   On-the-Go Breakfast Shake 19
   Flax Meal 21
   Banana Pancakes 23
   Breakfast Quiche 24
   Blueberry Muffins 25
   Breakfast Quesadilla 27
   Berry Breakfast Smoothie 29
   Scrambled Eggs and Chicken Sausage 30
   Fruit Parfait 32
   Almond Flour Waffles 34

LUNCH MEALS 36
   Chicken and Egg Salad 36
   Turkey Wrap 38
   Greek Blend Skewers 39
   Bean Burrito with a Kick 40
   Sweet Potato Casserole 42
   Salmon and Black Bean Salad 44
   Butternut Squash Soup 46
   Sweet Potato Nachos 48
   Veggie and Shrimp Rolls 50

- Broccoli with Toasted Almonds and Pepper 52
- Strawberry Graham Cracker Sandwich 54
- Avocado- Tomato Sandwich 55
- Chicken Peanut Butter Salad 56
- Eggplant Lasagna 58
- Chicken Caesar Salad Wrap 60

DINNER MEALS 62
- Vegetable Risotto 62
- Parmesan Chicken Pasta 64
- Classic Chicken with Carrots 66
- Sweet Chicken with Brussel Sprouts 68
- Steak Fajitas 70
- Roasted Chicken and Veggie Mix 72
- Sweet Apple Pork Chops 74
- Chicken Chili 76
- Zucchini Boats 78
- Loaded Peppers 80
- Kale Salad 82
- Cod Fillet 84
- Shrimp Potato Mix 86
- Turkey Meatloaf 88
- Cauliflower Mashed Potatoes 90

ABOUT THE AUTHOR 92
OTHER BOOKS 93
FREE BONUS 94

BREAKFAST MEALS

Oven- Baked Spinach and Tomato Omelet

This oven-baked omelet is a filling, healthy breakfast option that is full of rich, natural flavors. The spinach and tomato combination is perfect for an early morning breakfast.

Serves: 1 serving
Prep Time: 15 minutes
Cook Time: 20 minutes

Ingredients

- 1/2 cup of spinach
- 1/2 cup of chopped onion
- 4 grape tomatoes
- 3 egg whites

Directions:

1. Preheat oven to 425
2. Spray a medium sized skillet with cooking spray
3. Chop onion and tomato while oven is preheating
4. Sauté your chopped onion for 4 minutes on stove top then add your spinach and continue to sauté the mixture for 2 minutes
5. Place sautéed mixture into a medium sized bowl. Pour three egg whites over the mixture then add your sliced tomato
6. Pour mixture into your medium sized skillet and place in oven once oven is preheated.
7. Let bake for 20 minutes.

Nutritional Facts Per Serving:
Calories: 70
Total Fat: 0 g
Cholesterol 0 mg
Sodium 192mg
Carbohydrates: 3.7g
Protein 11.7g
Fiber 1g

Turnip Breakfast a Notch

This recipe adds a healthy twist to the classic breakfast potato. Your plate will be full of warm delicious goodness once the turnip finishes cooking.

Serves: 1 serving
Prep Time: 8 mins
Cook Time: 11 mins

Ingredients

- One turnip
- Pinch of black pepper
- Pinch of onion powder
- Tablespoon of olive oil

Directions

1. Peel and cut turnip into roughly 1-inch sized pieces then put them in a bowl and toss then with one tablespoon of olive oil. Add a pinch of black pepper and a pinch of onion powder.
2. Spray medium sized frying pan with non-stick spray.
3. Heat pan on stove top on medium.
4. Add turnip to pan and let cook on one side for 6 minutes. Then flip them and let cook for another 5 minutes until golden brown.

Nutritional Facts Per Serving:
Calories 167
Total Fat: 14.2g
Cholesterol: 0g
Sodium: 80mg
Carbohydrates: 11.6g
Protein: 1.7g
Fiber: 3.3g

Egg Puff French Toast Twist

Enjoy this healthier alternative to classic French toast. Not only is this recipe quick and easy, but it's also deliciously satisfying.

Serves: 1
Prep Time: 7 minutes
Cook Time: None

Ingredients

- 2 egg whites
- 1 teaspoon of Stevia
- 2 ounces of cream cheese
- 1 tablespoon of sugar free syrup

Directions

1. Put the cream cheese in a standard single serving sized bowl. Then, in the microwave, soften the cream cheese for about 25 seconds.
2. Add two eggs and 1 teaspoon of Stevia to the bowl and stir until they are blended.
3. Microwave again for 50 seconds this time and then stir again until blended.
4. Microwave again for 2 minutes. Once done microwaving, flip the bowl over on a plate. (You may need to use a fork to help loosen your egg puff or it might just fall right out onto the plate)
5. Top with tablespoon of sugar free syrup.

Nutritional Facts Per Serving:
Calories: 283
Total Fat: 19.2g
Cholesterol: 58mg
Sodium: 298mg
Carbohydrates: 7.1g
Protein: 9.7g
Fiber: 0.05g

Breakfast Ball Sandwich

These breakfast balls are a healthier way to enjoy a classic breakfast sandwich. The rich sausage and cheese flavors will leave a great taste in your mouth all morning long.

Serves: 6 servings
Prep Time: 15 minutes
Cook Time: 30 minutes

Ingredients

- 6 sausage patties
- 2 eggs
- 2 cups shredded cheddar cheese
- 2 ounces of cream cheese
- 1 cup almond flour

Directions

1. Preheat oven to 400
2. Add 2 cups of shredded cheddar cheese and cream cheese to bowl and microwave for 1 minute. Once mixture is softened stir together until combined.
3. In another medium bowl beat eggs and then add almond flour, leaving a small amount for step four. Add the cheese mixture from step one. Mix until fully combined.
4. Using the left over almond flour ball the dough into 6 even balls and place them on a plate then refrigerate until the balls are firm.

5. Flatten dough balls and place a sausage patty in the middle of each dough ball. Then add cream cheese on top of the sausage. Wrap the dough around sausage and cheese.
6. Grease muffin tin and put each doughball into separate muffin tin.
7. Bake for 15 minutes.

Nutritional Facts Per Serving:
Calories: 392
Total Fat: 29.16g
Cholesterol: 100mg
Sodium: 490mg
Carbohydrates: 8.3g
Protein:24.96g
Fiber: 3.3g

Avocado Breakfast Burrito

Jam-packed with all of the rich breakfast burrito flavors you love, this breakfast burrito won't leave you feeling sluggish. Instead you'll feel energized by the avocado, egg, and bacon bliss.

Serves: 1 serving
Prep Time: 15 minutes
Cook Time: 12 minutes

Ingredients

- 1 egg white
- 2 tablespoon of skim milk
- 2 slices of tomato
- 1/5 avocado
- 2 turkey bacon strips

Directions

1. Mix 1 egg and 2 tablespoons of milk
2. Spray frying pan with nonstick spray and heat to medium heat on stovetop
3. Add egg and milk mixture to pan
4. Let cook for about a minute or until done
5. Once crepe is solid flip to other side and let cook for an additional minute.
6. Once done add avocado, tomato, and turkey bacon. Roll it and use toothpick to hold wrap in place if necessary.

Nutritional Facts Per Serving:
Calories: 200
Total Fat: 15.2g
Cholesterol: 31mg
Sodium: 370mg
Carbohydrates: 8g
Protein: 20.5g
Fiber: 3.1g

On-the-Go Breakfast Shake

This protein packed option is great for on-the-move individuals. It's loaded up with healthy fuel for your body. And best of all, the shake can be ready in 5 minutes or less.

Serves: 1 serving
Prep Time: 5 minutes
Cook Time: Served cold

Ingredients:

- One whole banana
- 1 cup of plain non-fat yogurt
- 1/4 cup of blueberries
- 1/2 cup of ice
- Tablespoon of cool whip

Directions:

1. Slice banana
2. Blend one cup of plain non-fat yogurt with 1/4 cup of blueberries and banana
3. Add 1/2 cup of ice and continue to blend until smooth
4. Pour into cup
5. Add tablespoon of cool whip to top

Nutritional Facts Per Serving:
Calories: 269
Total Fat: 2.4g
Cholesterol: 0 mg
Sodium: 150mg
Carbohydrates: 55 g
Protein: 13.3g
Fiber: 5.1g

Flax Meal

Forget the old-fashioned oatmeal you're used to. This flax meal is bursting with those classic oatmeal flavors, including vanilla and cinnamon, but with half the carbs. The blueberries add a bit of sweetness.

Serves: 3
Prep Time 7 minutes
Cook Time: 8 minutes

Ingredients:

- 1 teaspoon cinnamon
- 1/4 cup of fresh blueberries
- 1 1/2 cup of almond milk
- 2 tablespoons of flaxseed meal
- 1 teaspoon of vanilla extract
- 1 cup of almond flour

Directions

1. Warm medium pot on stovetop at medium heat.
2. Combine cinnamon, flaxseed meal, and almond flour in medium bowl.
3. Pour almond milk and vanilla into medium pot on stovetop then add the dry combined ingredients.
4. Cook for 8 minutes stirring the entire time with a whisk. Add vanilla at 6 minutes.
5. Once thick it is ready to serve. Add blueberries to the top before serving.

Nutritional Facts Per Serving:
Calories: 295
Total Fat: 21.42g
Cholesterol: 0mg
Sodium: 76mg
Carbohydrates: 15.87g
Protein: 9.7g
Fiber: 7.3g

Banana Pancakes

Banana flavored pancakes are a naturally sweet option for breakfast. Topped with syrup, this is a classic breakfast choice.

Serves: 1 serving
Prep Time: 5 minutes
Cook Time: 2 minutes

Ingredients

- 2 egg whites
- 1 banana
- 2 tablespoons sugar free syrup

Directions

1. Whisk eggs
2. Mash banana after peeling
3. Mix egg and mashed banana
4. Spray medium pan with non-stick and heat on medium
5. Pour two pancakes and cook for a minute on each side or until golden
6. Pour sugar free syrup over top and serve

Nutritional Facts Per Serving:
Calories: 229
Total Fat: 8.6g
Cholesterol: 0mg
Sodium: 230mg
Carbohydrates: 31.8g
Protein: 13.9g
Fiber: 3.1g

Breakfast Quiche

Full of natural veggies and ham, this breakfast quiche is mouth-wateringly wonderful.

Serves: 1
Prep Time: 10 minutes
Cook Time: 20 minutes

Ingredients

- 2 egg whites
- 1 tablespoon of milk
- 1/8 cup chopped onion
- 1/8 cup chopped green pepper
- 1/8 cup ham
- 1/8 cup shredded cheddar cheese

Directions

1. Preheat oven to 400 degrees
2. Chop onion, green pepper, and ham
3. In medium bowl combine eggs and milk. Whisk together
4. Add onion, green pepper, ham, and cheese
5. Pour into a ramekin and let bake for about 20 minutes or until done

Nutritional Facts Per Serving:
Calories: 268
Total Fat: 20.48g
Cholesterol: 32mg
Sodium: 80mg
Carbohydrates: 4.96g
Protein: 19.81g
Fiber: 0.58g

Blueberry Muffins

These scrumptious, fluffy, warm muffins will make your mouth water before they even get out of the oven. Your whole family will be excited to try these delicious muffins.

Serves: 12
Prep Time: 10 minutes
Cook Time: 25 minutes

Ingredients

- 1 cup almond flour
- 2 egg whites
- 1 cup oats
- 1/2 cup coconut sugar
- 1/2 cup water
- 1 teaspoon baking soda
- 1/2 cup applesauce (unsweetened)
- 1 teaspoon cinnamon
- 1 cup frozen blueberries

Directions

1. Preheat oven to 350 and spray a 12-cup muffin tin with nonstick spray.
2. Mix almond flour, baking soda, oats, and cinnamon.
3. Add applesauce, egg whites, sugar, and water. Mix until completely blended.
4. Mix in blueberries last.
5. Pour into muffin tin and bake for 25 minutes or until done.

Nutritional Facts Per Serving:
Calories: 109.91
Total Fat: 5g
Cholesterol: 0g
Sodium: 134mg
Carbohydrates: 14.5g
Protein: 3.16g
Fiber: 2.21g

Breakfast Quesadilla

This crispy, going quesadilla is packed with cheddar cheese, bacon and salsa. What a great way to kick off your morning on a high note.

Serves 2
Prep Time: 10 minutes
Cook Time: 5 minutes

Ingredients

- 2 egg whites
- 1/8 cup of shredded cheddar cheese
- 1 turkey bacon strip (diced)
- 1/8 cup of salsa
- 2 whole wheat tortillas (8 inches)

Directions

1. In a small bowl whisk egg whites
2. Spray medium pan with nonstick spray and heat on medium
3. Scramble egg mixture in pan and then put in a bowl when done
4. Add first tortilla to pan and top with half of the cheese, bacon, and egg. Let cook for 3 minutes or until brown
5. Repeat with second tortilla
6. Serve with salsa

Nutritional Facts Per Serving:
Calories: 194.5
Total Fat 6.5g
Cholesterol 13mg
Sodium 340mg
Carbohydrates 27.42g
Protein 23.3g
Fiber 3.13

Berry Breakfast Smoothie

This berry smoothie is a great way to start your day off right. The healthy spinach taste is hidden by the berry banana flavors. This is an easy way to get some veggies before noon.

Serves: 1
Prep Time: 5 minutes
Cook Time: NA

Ingredients

- 1/2 cup frozen spinach
- 1/4 cup frozen assorted berries
- 1 banana
- 1/4 cup water

Directions

1. Combine all ingredients in blender and blend until smooth (typically 1 to two minutes)
2. Enjoy!

Nutritional Facts Per Serving:
Calories: 140
Total Fat: 0.45g
Cholesterol: 0mg
Sodium: 48mg
Carbohydrates: 34mg
Protein: 3.7g
Fiber: 7.4g

Scrambled Eggs and Chicken Sausage

This timeless breakfast combo is full of tasty flavors, including sausage and fresh spinach, but with half of the calories. The scrambled eggs are fluffy and delicious too, which pair perfectly with the rich taste of the sausage.

Serves: 1
Prep Time: 10 minutes
Cook Time: 15 minutes

Ingredients:

- 3 egg whites
- 1/4 cup almond milk
- 3.3 ounces chicken apple sausage diced
- Pinch of salt
- Pinch of pepper
- 1/2 cup fresh spinach
- Tablespoon of olive oil

Directions:

1. Heat 2 medium sized frying pans
2. Dice chicken sausage into quarter sized pieces
3. Whisk eggs, milk, pepper, and salt together in a bowl
4. In a separate bowl toss spinach in the olive oil
5. Pour egg, milk, pepper, salt mix into frying pan and stir lightly so eggs stay fluffy (Should take about 5 minutes)
6. While eggs are cooking in a separate frying pan cook diced sausage. Sausage should take about 6 minutes

on medium or until golden brown. Throw the spinach in with the sausage the last couple minutes of cook time and mix together.
7. Remove sausage/ spinach mix and serve on side of scrambled eggs.

Nutritional Facts Per Serving:
Calories: 294
Total Fat: 18.6g
Cholesterol: 68mg
Sodium: 759mg
Carbohydrates: 1.7g
Protein: 30.9g
Fiber: 0.7g

Fruit Parfait

This fruity mix is a perfect morning treat. The berries and granola make the protein-rich Greek yogurt flavorful and crunchy.

Serves 2
Prep Time: 10 minutes
Cook Time: NA

Ingredients:

- 1 banana
- 1/4 cup blue berries
- 1/4 cup blackberries
- 5 large strawberries
- 1 cup vanilla Greek yogurt
- 1/8 cup Granola

Directions:

1. Slice banana into quarter inch wide pieces and put in medium size bowl
2. Cut strawberries down the middle into two even piece then put in with banana
3. Add blue berries and blackberries to bowl
4. Mix yogurt in last
5. Sprinkle granola over the top
6. Serve and enjoy!

Nutritional Facts Per Serving:
Calories: 215
Total Fat: 2.25g
Cholesterol: 6mg
Sodium: 84mg
Carbohydrates: 43.35g
Protein: 7.5g
Fiber: 4.5g

Almond Flour Waffles

This comfort food can be enjoyed the healthy way. The slight nutty undertones of the waffles will appeal to a broad audience.

Serves: 8
Prep Time: 5 minutes
Cook Time: 20 minutes

Ingredients:

- 1 cup almond flour
- 1 pinch salt
- 1 teaspoon baking soda
- 4 eggs
- 1/4 cup honey
- 1 teaspoon vanilla

Directions:

1. Preheat waffle iron for a few minutes and spray it with nonstick spray
2. Combine the salt, almond flour, and baking soda in a medium bowl
3. In another medium bowl, combine honey, eggs, and vanilla
4. Combine both mixtures
5. Spoon batter out onto the iron and continue cooking until each waffle is golden brown

Nutritional Facts Per Serving:
Calories: 181.5
Total Fat: 10g
Cholesterol: 88mg
Sodium: 157mg
Carbohydrates: 20.56g
Protein: 5.7g
Fiber: 1.7g

LUNCH MEALS

Chicken and Egg Salad

This chicken and egg salad has a pleasant kick to it. It works well as a lunch pick-me-up. It has a creamy texture that you'll love.

Serves: 4
Prep Time: 1 hour
Cook Time: 20 minutes

Ingredients:

- 2 medium chicken breasts
- 3 eggs hardboiled
- 2 tablespoons of fat-free mayo
- 1 tablespoon of curry powder

Directions:

1. Preheat oven to 360F
2. Cook the chicken breast in the oven for 20 minutes
3. Boil water over the stovetop and place eggs in water for 8 minutes until they are hardboiled
4. Mix mayo and curry powder in small bowl
5. Cut the chicken and eggs into small pieces and mix them into the mayo/curry mix
6. Put mixture in the fridge for 30 minutes so it is cool to serve

Nutritional Facts Per Serving:
Calories: 175
Total Fat: 5.4g
Cholesterol: 180 mg
Sodium: 152mg
Carbohydrates: 1.6g
Protein: 30g
Fiber: 0.8g

Turkey Wrap

This cool and satisfying wrap makes for a delicious lunch option. Exploding with feta and humus flavoring, this wrap doesn't disappoint.

Serves: 1
Prep Time: 10 minutes
Cook Time: NA

Ingredients:

- 1/4 cup of sliced turkey
- 1/4 cup of cucumber
- 1/4 cup of diced tomato
- 1/4 cup feta cheese
- 1 tablespoons of humus
- 1 whole wheat wrap

Directions:

1. Dice tomato, cut cucumber, and cut turkey
2. Spread 1 tablespoon of humus onto whole wheat wrap
3. Sprinkle feta cheese, cucumber, diced tomato, and sliced turkey onto wrap and fold

Nutritional Facts Per Serving:
Calories: 270
Total Fat: 7g
Cholesterol: 40mg
Sodium: 580mg
Carbohydrates: 28g
Protein: 36g
Fiber: 11g

Greek Blend Skewers

These skewers are a fun and filling lunch option that will bring a little extra flavor to your day. You can always add on chicken, lamb or beef chunks to the skewers for extra protein without any additional carbs.

Serves: 12
Prep Time: 10 minutes
Cook Time: NA

Ingredients:

- 3 ounces of 1/2 inch cubes of feta cheese (about 12 cubes)
- 12 green olives
- 12 cherry tomatoes
- 1/4 cup of Greek salad dressing (low fat)
- 12 slices of cucumber

Directions:

1. Skewer 1 olive, 1 tomato, I cucumber slice, and one cube of cheese
2. Drizzle low fat Greek dressing over skewers

Nutritional Facts Per Serving:
Calories: 55
Total Fat: 5g
Cholesterol: 6mg
Sodium: 150mg
Carbohydrates: 3g
Protein: 1g
Fiber: 1g

Bean Burrito with a Kick

Protein packed and full of flavor, this hardy, filling option will keep you going on your busiest of days. This burrito is jam-packed with favors that will make your mouth water.

Serves: 1
Prep Time: 10 mins.
Cook Time: NA

Ingredients:

- 1 tortilla (whole wheat)
- 1/2 cup romaine lettuce chopped
- 1/4 cup refried beans
- 1 tablespoon jalapenos
- 1/4 cup chopped cherry tomatoes
- 1 scallion chopped
- 2 tablespoons Greek yogurt, nonfat and plain preferred
- 2 tablespoons shredded cheese

Directions:

1. Chop cherry tomatoes, scallion, and romaine lettuce
2. Lay out tortilla and fill it with lettuce, beans, jalapenos, tomato, scallion, yogurt and cheese
3. Wrap burrito

Nutritional Facts Per Serving:
Calories: 270
Total Fat: 9g
Cholesterol: 15mg
Sodium: 570mg
Carbohydrates: 33g
Protein: 14.1g
Fiber: 9g

Sweet Potato Casserole

Golden, fluffy, and full of sweet flavors, this casserole is a must try. It's like dessert for lunch, but much healthier.

Serves: 10
Prep Time:30 minutes
Cook Time: 12 minutes

Ingredients:

- Pinch of pepper
- Pinch of cinnamon
- 3/4 cup of marshmallows (mini kind works best)
- 1/4 cup toasted pecans
- 3 tablespoons butter
- 2 tablespoons brown sugar
- 4 medium sized sweet potatoes peeled and cut into 1-inch pieces

Directions:

1. Melt butter in microwave for 40 seconds until completely melted
2. Chop pecans into small pieces
3. Peel and cut sweet potatoes into small pieces (about an inch)
4. Pour a single cup of water in a multicooker
5. With handles up place a trivet into the multicooker
6. Put in sweet potatoes then close the lid and cook with pressure on high for 12 minutes

7. Lift the trivet to drain the water
8. Place potatoes back in the multicooker and then combine the cinnamon, nutmeg, butter, vanilla, brown sugar, pinch of salt and pepper by stirring
9. Use the marshmallows and pecans to top

Nutritional Facts Per Serving:
Calories: 190
Total Fat: 6g
Cholesterol: 9mg
Sodium: 190mg
Carbohydrates: 33g
Protein: 2.1g
Fiber: 3.8g

Salmon and Black Bean Salad

This nutrient packed, refreshing salad is full of healthy ingredients that will give you extra energy all afternoon. The rich, creamy flavor won't disappoint.

Serves: 1
Prep time: 10 minutes
Cook time: 15 minutes

Ingredients
- 1 4-ounce salmon
- 1/2 cup of canned black beans
- 1/2 cup of cherry tomatoes
- 1 teaspoon of olive oil
- 1/2 avocado
- 1 pinch of cumin
- 1 pinch of salt
- 1 pinch of pepper
- 1 cup of spinach

Directions
1. Preheat oven to 425
2. Bake salmon for 10-15 minutes or until it is easily flaked
3. While salmon is baking dice avocado and tomatoes
4. In serving bowl put spinach at bottom for salad. Throw avocado, tomatoes and salmon over top. Last, sprinkle cumin, salt, pepper, and olive oil over the top

Nutritional Facts Per Serving:
Calories: 521
Fat: 24.5g
Cholesterol: 71mg
Carb: 29g
sodium: 669mg
Protein: 35g
Fiber: 20.1g

Butternut Squash Soup

This warm and creamy lunch option is a soothing midday treat. The butternut squash flavor is a delicious option for any time of the year.

Serves: 6
Prep time: 10 minutes
Cook time: 40 minutes

Ingredients:
- 3 cups of vegetable broth (low-sodium type)
- 2 teaspoons canola
- Pinch of nutmeg
- 2 shallot
- 1 butternut squash
- 1/4 cup of half and half (fat-free)

Directions:
1. Heat oil in pressure cook
2. Chop shallot and put them in pressure cooker for a couple minutes while you peel your butternut squash and cube
3. Add squash, broth, and nutmeg to pressure cooker for about 20 minutes and continue on high. After 20 minutes release and let sit for 10 minutes.
4. Use blend to purée mixer. Depending on what size blender you own you might have to do this in parts.
5. Put soup back in the pressure cooker and stir in half and half. Leave on medium heat for 3 minutes.

Nutritional Facts Per Serving:
Calories: 60
Fat: 1.5g
Cholesterol: 0mg
Carb: 12g
Sodium: 126mg
Protein: 2g
Fiber: 2g

Sweet Potato Nachos

These crunchy and filling nachos are a healthy option for nacho lovers. This is also a wonderful party appetizer.

Serves: 4
Prep time: 10 minutes
Cook time: 20 minutes

Ingredients:
- 2 pounds of sweet potatoes
- 1 tablespoon oil
- 1/3 cup of canned black beans
- 1/3 cup of shredded Mexican cheese
- 1/2 cup of tomatoes
- 1/3 cup of avocado
- 1 teaspoon of Mexican seasoning mix of choice

Directions:
1. Preheat oven to 400
2. Spray cooking spray with nonstick
3. Slice potatoes very thinly after peeling then lay them out on tray
4. Spread oil over top evenly along with the seasoning mix.
5. Bake for 10 minutes in the oven and then flip and bake for another 10 minutes until crisp
6. Remove pan and immediately sprinkle cheese. Then sprinkling the beans and avocado.
7. Serve hot

Calories: 313
Fat: 8.25g
Cholesterol: 7.5mg
Carbs: 48g
Sodium: 291mg
Protein: 9g
Fiber: 9g

Veggie and Shrimp Rolls

These refreshing rolls have an appealing crunch to it. They are bursting with a medley of vegetable flavors that pair perfectly with the peanut butter.

Serves: 4
Prep time: 10 minutes
Cook time: 5 minutes

Ingredients:
- 3 ounces of shrimp
- 4 rice paper wraps
- 1 cucumber
- 1 carrot
- 1 zucchini
- 3 lettuce leaves (iceberg)
- 4 cups of water
- 2 tablespoons of peanut butter

Directions:
1. Place medium pan on stove top at a boil
2. Peel cucumber, carrot, and zucchini and cut into thin pieces the long way
3. Peel and drain shrimp
4. Boil shrimp for 5 minutes or until done. Strain and put in a bowl in the fridge to cool.
5. Spread peanut butter evenly on four wraps.
6. Place cucumber, carrot, and zucchini evenly on four wraps.
7. Last add shrimp evenly onto four wraps.
8. Roll and enjoy!

Nutritional Facts Per Serving:
Calories: 213
Fat: 6.8g
Cholesterol: 50mg
Sodium: 201mg
Carbs: 23g
Protein: 12.5g
Fiber: 4.2g

Broccoli with Toasted Almonds and Pepper

Full of ginger and soy sauce, this lunch option will satisfy your appetite for the rest of the afternoon. The crushed red pepper adds a pleasant kick.

Serves: 3
Prep Time: 10
Cook Time: 10

Ingredients:

- 4 cups of broccoli
- 1 tablespoons of toast almonds (buy the prep sliced)
- 1 teaspoons of low-sodium soy sauce
- 1 pinch of ginger
- 1 pinch of crushed red pepper
- 1 tablespoon of dried roast red pepper

Directions:

1. Boil water on the stovetop
2. Trim broccoli to make bite sized pieces then boil for 8 minutes
3. Chop the ginger finely
4. In a small bowl mix red pepper, toasted almonds, soy sauce, and ginger
5. Strain broccoli when done and then pour mixture over top of broccoli

Nutritional Facts Per Serving:
Calories: 75
Total Fat: 4g
Cholesterol: 0mg
Sodium: 120mg
Carbohydrates: 9g
Protein: 4.2g
Fiber: 4.1g

Strawberry Graham Cracker Sandwich

This dessert-fo- lunch option will make you feel like you're splurging with your calories when, in fact, you're eating healthily. Strawberry lovers will be in heaven with this recipe.

Serves: 2
Prep Time: 5 minutes
Cook Time: NA

Ingredients:

- 2 Graham crackers
- 4 strawberries
- 2 tablespoons of light strawberry cream cheese

Directions:

1. Slice the strawberries thinly
2. Break Graham Crackers in half to create 4 crackers
3. Spread cream cheese on graham crackers
4. Place strawberries in the middle to make two sandwiches

Nutritional Facts Per Serving:
Calories: 250
Total Fat: 8g
Cholesterol: 16mg
Sodium: 400mg
Carbohydrates: 38g
Protein: 6g
Fiber: 2g

Avocado- Tomato Sandwich

Creamy avocado and tasty tomato make this a delicious option for a light lunch. Fresh tastes will explode in your mouth with this open-faced sandwich.

Serves 1
Prep Time: 5 minutes
Cook Time: N/A

Ingredients:

- Slice of tomato
- 1/4 avocado
- Pinch of salt
- Pinch of pepper
- 1 piece of whole grain bread
-

Directions:

1. Toast whole grain bread in the toaster until golden brown
2. Mash avocado then spread it on piece of toast
3. Place tomato slice of the top of toast
4. Sprinkle pepper and salt over top

Nutritional Facts Per Serving:
Calories: 151
Total Fat: 9.2g
Cholesterol: 0mg
Sodium: 152mg
Carbohydrates: 14.5g
Protein: 3.8g
Fiber: 2.1g

Chicken Peanut Butter Salad

This flavorful salad is rich in taste. You will feel definitely full until dinnertime.

Serves: 1
Prep time: 10 minutes
Cook time: 10 minutes

Ingredients:

- 1 tsp curry powder
- 1 pinch of cumin
- 1 chicken breast fillet
- 1 tablespoon smooth peanut butter
- 1 tablespoon of lemon juice
- 1/4 cucumber
- 1/2 iceberg lettuce wedge

Directions:

1. Grease pan with nonstick spray and heat to medium heat on stovetop
2. Cut chicken breast into thin long strips and cook on stove top until done (about 4 minutes on each side)
3. Heat peanut butter for 20 seconds
4. Mix lemon juice, peanut butter, curry powder, and cumin in small bowl
5. Chop cucumber into small pieces
6. Chop iceberg lettuce and place in serving bowl
7. Put chicken and cucumber in serving bowl and then pour mixture evenly over
8. Serve

Nutritional Facts Per Serving:
Calories: 246
Total Fat: 11.85g
Cholesterol: 90mg
Sodium: 248mg
Carbohydrates: 9.2g
Protein: 30.65g
Fiber: 4g

Eggplant Lasagna

This eggplant lasagna is a healthy twist on the classic. Full of new and old flavors, you'll love this nutrient-rich alternative.

Serves: 6
Prep Time: 10 minutes
Cook Time: 6 hours

Ingredients:

- 2 eggplants
- 1 cup mozzarella cheese (low-fat)
- 24 ounces spaghetti sauce (low-fat)
- 1 bell pepper
- 1 onion
- 1 cup cottage cheese (low-fat)
- 1 egg white

Directions:

1. Peel and slice eggplants thinly (lasagna noodle sized)
2. Chop onion and bell pepper into small pieces
3. Combine cottage cheese, egg white, and mozzarella
4. Pour 6 ounces of spaghetti sauce into your slow cooker
5. Lay 1/4 eggplant slices evenly along bottom of slow cooker then cover with 1/4 of the onions, bell pepper and cheese mix (repeat to make 3 layers)
6. Set slow cooker to low and let cook for 6 hours
7. Serve hot

Nutritional Facts Per Serving:
Calories: 220
Total Fat: 10.5g
Cholesterol: 60mg
Sodium: 765mg
Carbohydrates: 19g
Protein: 13.8g
Fiber: 3.5g

Chicken Caesar Salad Wrap

This hands-free meal is good for meals on-the-run. The chicken caesar salad recipe will fill you up with its classic flavor.

Serves: 2
Prep Time: 10 minutes
Cook Time: 15 minutes

Ingredients:

- 1 chicken breast
- 2 spinach tortillas
- 1 tablespoon shredded parmesan cheese (low-cal)
- 1 cup romaine lettuce
- 1 tablespoon olive oil
- 1 tablespoon of Caesar salad dressing (low-cal)

Directions:

1. Cut chicken breast into thin even strips
2. Grease pan with nonstick spray
3. Cook chicken on stove top for about 5 minutes on each side on medium heat or until done
4. Lay out tortillas and spread lettuce evenly between both wraps
5. Lay chicken evenly between both wraps on top of lettuce then sprinkle with cheese, Caesar salad dressing and oil
6. Roll wrap and serve

Nutritional Facts Per Serving:
Calories: 467
Total Fat: 18.5g
Cholesterol: 50mg
Sodium: 567mg
Carbohydrates: 84mg
Protein: 19.1g
Fiber: 7g

DINNER MEALS

Vegetable Risotto

This risotto dish, which is packed with garlic, cheese, sage, and squash, makes a truly delicious dinner choice. Enjoy this hearty, guilt-free meal.

Serves: 8
Prep Time: 10 minutes
Cook Time: 3 hours

Ingredients:

- 2 tablespoons vegetable oil
- 4 cups vegetable broth (low-sodium type)
- 1 1/4 cup Arborio rice
- 1/4 cup of shredded cheese of choice (low-fat)
- 2 cups butternut squash
- 1 pinch of garlic powder
- 1 pinch of sage
- 1 small onion

Directions:

1. Cube butternut squash
2. Chop onion into small pieces
3. Mix vegetable oil, broth, rice, butternut squash, garlic powder, sage, and onion into slow cooker
4. Cook on high for 3 hours or until the rice is done and most of the liquid has been absorbed
5. Last mix in the cheese and then serve hot

Nutritional Facts Per Serving:
Calories: 180
Total Fat: 5.1g
Cholesterol: 1.5mg
Sodium: 70mg
Carbohydrates: 31g
Protein: 4.1g
Fiber: 2g

Parmesan Chicken Pasta

This classic chicken and pasta dish has a wonderful cheesy, garlic flavor, which is enjoyed any night of the week.

Serves:4
Prep Time:15 minutes
Cook Time: 30 minutes\

Ingredients:

- 8 ounces penne pasta (gluten free)
- 2 tablespoons olive oil
- 2 large chicken breasts
- 1 pinch of salt
- 1 pinch of pepper
- 4 cloves of garlic
- 1 bag of spinach (fresh not frozen)
- 1/2 cup white wine
- 1 teaspoon of lemon juice
- 1/8 cup of shredded parmesan cheese

Directions:

1. Boil pasta on stovetop then strain when done
2. Mince garlic cloves and chop spinach while pasta boils
3. Cut chicken into small pieces
4. Spray medium sized pan with nonstick
5. Season chicken with salt and pepper then cook on stove top over medium heat until done (10 minutes) keep chicken moving so no sides burn

6. Add garlic, wine, and lemon juice to pan and continue cooking for about 3 minutes
7. Remove from pan and put into a medium sized bowl. Mix in chopped spinach, olive oil and pasta.
8. Serve hot

Nutritional Facts Per Serving:
Calories: 340
Total Fat: 12g
Cholesterol: 70mg
Sodium: 500mg
Carbohydrates: 24g
Protein: 30g
Fiber: 2.1g

Classic Chicken with Carrots

This simple chicken dish is extremely favorful. Dinner has never been so easy, yet satisfying.

Serves: 1
Prep Time: 10 minutes
Cook Time: 1 hour

Ingredients:

- 1 cup baby carrots
- 1 medium chicken breast
- 1 pinch of sage
- 1 pinch of salt
- 1 pinch of pepper
- Tablespoon of butter

Directions:

1. Preheat oven to 450
2. Sprinkle pepper and salt over chicken breast
3. Cook on baking sheet for 35 minutes or until done
4. While chicken is cooking put carrots into medium sized pan and add about a cup of water and a pinch of sage. Bring the water to a boil then cover the pan and turn down to medium-low. Let sit for about 20 minutes or until carrots are tender.
5. Drain the carrots and then toss with the butter

Nutritional Facts Per Serving:
Calories: 353
Total Fat: 17g
Cholesterol: 130mg
Sodium: 356mg
Carbohydrates: 20.3g
Protein: 32.1g
Fiber: 7.1g

Sweet Chicken with Brussel Sprouts

Bursting with flavor, this chicken recipe is sweet and delicious. If you like apples this is the recipe for you. The brussel sprouts are the perfect side to this healthy option.

Serves 4
Prep Time: 20
Cook Time: 15

Ingredients:

- 2 tablespoons olive oil
- 3 tablespoons red wine vinegar
- 2 tablespoons light syrup
- 1 cup Brussels sprouts
- 1/4 cup dried currants
- 1 apple
- 4 chicken breasts
- 1 pinch of salt
- 1 pinch of pepper

Directions:

1. Cut apple into slices
2. Slice chicken breasts into two pieces
3. Heat a large pan on stovetop over medium heat after spraying with nonstick spray
4. Season chicken pieces with pepper and salt

5. Add chicken and one tablespoon of oil to pan and cook for about 4 minutes on both sides or until they appear done
6. Remove from pan and place in a separate bowl
7. Add 2 tablespoons of vinegar and syrup to the pan and cook for about a minute then return chicken to the pan and turn it over to evenly coat in the glaze
8. Slice brussels sprouts in half
9. Mix 1 tablespoon oil, 1 tablespoon vinegar in large bowl then add brussels sprouts, apple, and currants to bowl and mix
10. Heat in pan for 2 minutes on stovetop
11. Serve with chicken

Nutritional Facts Per Serving:
Calories: 290
Total Fat: 8.7g
Cholesterol: 59mg
Sodium: 290mg
Carbohydrates: 23g
Protein: 28g
Fiber: 4g

Steak Fajitas

These fajitas deliver a mouthwatering blend of flavor. This delicious mix of steak and vegetables will be enjoyed by the whole family.

Serves:2
Prep Time: 10 minutes
Cook Time: 6 hours

Ingredients:

- 2 ounces of steak
- 1 onion
- 1 green bell pepper
- 1 yellow bell pepper
- 1 red bell pepper
- 1 package of taco seasoning
- 1/4 cup of water

Directions:
1. Slice steak into small chunks
2. Slice peppers and chop onion into small pieces
3. Place onions into slow cooker first to layer the bottom
4. Rub the steak in the taco seasoning and place over onions
5. Place peppers over top of chicken last
6. Last, add water
7. Cook on high for 6 hours or until done

Nutritional Facts Per Serving:
Calories: 137.5
Total Fat: 2g
Cholesterol: 45mg
Sodium: 205mg
Carbohydrates: 17g
Protein: 15g
Fiber: 2.5g

Roasted Chicken and Veggie Mix

This moist chicken recipe is an easy dinner option. It is packed with enjoyable flavors, including paprika and natural veggies.

Serves: 2
Prep Time: 10 minutes
Cook Time: 15 minutes

Ingredients:

- 2 medium chicken breasts
- 1 bell pepper
- 1 zucchini
- 1 cup of broccoli
- 1 tomato
- 2 tablespoons of olive oil
- 1 pinch of salt
- 1 pinch of pepper
- 1 pinch of paprika

Directions:

1. Preheat oven to 475
2. Chop vegetables into medium pieces (bell pepper, zucchini, broccoli, tomato)
3. Chop chicken into cubes
4. Spray baking pan with nonstick spray
5. Combine vegetables, chicken, pepper, salt, olive oil and paprika in large bowl then spread out in baking pan
6. Bake for about 15 minutes or until chicken is done

Nutritional Facts Per Serving:
Calories: 250
Total Fat: 15g
Cholesterol: 55mg
Sodium: 350mg
Carbohydrates: 6.2g
Protein: 20g
Fiber: 1.5g

Sweet Apple Pork Chops

This salty and sweet combination is a deliciously healthy dinner option that the whole family will enjoy.

Serves: 4
Prep Time: 10
Cook Time: 20

Ingredients:

- 3 medium pork chops
- 2 tablespoons olive oil
- 3/4 cup of chicken stock (low-sodium)
- 2 medium apples
- 1 red onion
- 1 teaspoon Dijon mustard

Directions:

1. Slice apples and onion thinly
2. Heat pan to medium high on stovetop. Add 1 tablespoon of olive oil and then add pork chops. Cook on each side for 5 minutes.
3. Mix chicken stock and mustard in a bowl while pork chops cook
4. Remove pork chops
5. Put sliced apples and sliced onion in pan with 1 tablespoon of olive oil. Continue stirring and let cook for about 5 minutes.

6. Pour stock/ mustard mixture into pan and then add pork chops back into pan
7. Cook for 4 minutes
8. Serve hot

Nutritional Facts Per Serving:
Calories: 350
Total Fat: 19g
Cholesterol: 96mg
Sodium: 340mg
Carbohydrates: 16g
Protein: 31g
Fiber: 17g

Chicken Chili

This chili recipe is a warm and yummy dinner option full of protein and flavor. Topped with cheesy goodness, this recipe is a low- calorie alternative to the hardy classic chili that we all love.

Serves: 3
Prep Time: 10 minutes
Cook Time: 25 minutes

Ingredients:

- 3 cups of chicken stock (low sodium)
- 2 cups of cooked shredded chicken
- 1 can of pinto beans
- 1 cup of salsa (low sodium)
- 1/8 cup shredded Mexican blend cheese

Directions:

1. Add chicken stock, shredded chicken, beans, and salsa to medium pot on stovetop
2. Stir and combine then heat over medium-high heat for about 15 minutes or until boil
3. Turn heat down to low and let cook for another 5 minutes
4. Pour into individual bowl and then top with cheese

Nutritional Facts Per Serving:
Calories: 404
Total Fat: 8.1g
Cholesterol: 111.1mg
Sodium: 611mg
Carbohydrates: 31.5g
Protein: 38g
Fiber: 8.5g

Zucchini Boats

This dinner option is great because not only is it full of flavor, but it's also fun! No matter your age, you'll surely enjoy eating your boat.

Serves: 2
Prep Time: 10 minutes
Cook Time: 20 minutes

Ingredients:

- 1 zucchini
- 1 tablespoon of olive oil
- 2 ounces of ground sausage
- 6 cherry tomatoes
- 1/8 cup shredded parmesan cheese

Directions:

1. Preheat oven to 350
2. Cut zucchini down the middle to make two even pieces then scoop out the middle and put into a separate bowl diced
3. Cut cherry tomatoes in half
4. Cook sausage in a medium pan on stovetop with olive oil on medium heat until done (8 minutes)
5. Add zucchini middle and tomatoes and continue cooking for 5 minutes
6. Spoon mixture into zucchini boats and top with cheese
7. Bake for 20 minutes

Nutritional Facts Per Serving:
Calories: 208
Total Fat: 16g
Cholesterol: 25mg
Sodium: 337.5mg
Carbohydrates: 7.5g
Protein: 9.5g
Fiber: 1.6g

Loaded Peppers

These loaded peppers are a healthy twist on classic stuffed peppers. Full of delicious flavors that are also great fuel for your body, this dinner will leave you feeling energized.

Serves: 2
Prep Time: 15 minutes
Cook Time: 30 minutes

Ingredients:

- 2 bell peppers
- 1 cup of cooked quinoa
- 1/2 cup of shredded pepper jack cheese
- 1/3 cup of salsa
- 1/3 pack of Morning Star black bean crumble

Directions:

1. Preheat oven to 350
2. Cut tops of bell peppers and remove cores
3. Cook the black bean crumble according to package directions
4. Mix crumble, quinoa, cheese, and salsa
5. Put mixture evenly into each pepper and then bake in over for 30 minutes

Nutritional Facts Per Serving:
Calories: 326
Total Fat: 12.5g
Cholesterol: 25mg
Sodium: 600mg
Carbohydrates: 35g
Protein: 19g
Fiber: 7.8g

Kale Salad

Who says that salad can't be lip-smackingly-good? This kale salad will leave you craving more.

Serves: 2
Prep Time: 10 minutes
Cook Time: 0

Ingredients:

- 1 bunch of kale
- 3 tablespoons of apple cider vinegar
- 1 tablespoon of soy sauce (low sodium)
- 1 tablespoon maple syrup (sugar free)
- 1 tablespoon almond butter
- 6 cherry tomatoes

Directions:

1. Wash kale and then chop it into pieces
2. Cut cherry tomatoes in half and mix in large bowl with kale
3. Mix soy sauce, vinegar, syrup, and almond butter together
4. Pour mixture over kale and cherry tomatoes then toss kale and cherry tomato in mixture

Nutritional Facts Per Serving:
Calories: 109
Total Fat: 5g
Cholesterol: 0g
Sodium: 440mg
Carbohydrates: 12g
Protein: 3g
Fiber: 1.3g

Cod Fillet

This pleasingly flakey fillet is perfect for dinner. With its soy and ginger essence, it won't disappoint.

Serves: 4
Prep Time: 10 minutes
Cook Time: 10 minutes

Ingredients:

- 3 tablespoons vinegar
- Pinch of salt
- Pinch of pepper
- Tablespoon of soy sauce (low sodium)
- 4 skinless cod fillets
- 2 tablespoons of grated ginger
- 4 scallions

Directions:

1. Grease a medium sized pan with nonstick spray
2. Combine vinegar, soy sauce, and ginger in a bowl
3. Season cod fillets with pepper and salt then place in pan with vinegar, soy sauce, ginger combination
4. Cook on medium heat until fish is thoroughly cooked (about 10 minutes)
5. Cut scallions into small pieces and then sprinkle over fish in pan
6. Serve

Nutritional Facts Per Serving:
Calories: 114.5
Total Fat: 1.5g
Cholesterol: 18.7mg
Sodium: 244mg
Carbohydrates: 1.2g
Protein: 7.8g
Fiber: .1g

Shrimp Potato Mix

This filling combination has an enjoyable kick to it that you'll fall in love with. Great for anyone who likes a little bit of spice.

Serves: 4
Prep Time: 10
Cook Time: 20

Ingredients:

- 2 tablespoons olive oil
- 4 potatoes
- 2 scallions
- 1/2 pound of shrimp
- 1 pinch of curry powder

Directions:

1. Wash, skin, and dice potatoes
2. Chop scallions into small pieces
3. Devein and peel shrimp
4. Spray medium sized pan and heat on medium. Cook potatoes and olive oil for 12 minutes over stovetop.
5. Add scallions to pan and cook for an additional minute
6. Add shrimp and curry powder to pan and cook for an additional 5 minutes

Nutritional Facts Per Serving:
Calories: 260
Total Fat:8.8g
Cholesterol: 111.3mg
Sodium: 176.3mg
Carbohydrates: 19.5g
Protein: 25g
Fiber: 1.9g

Turkey Meatloaf

This savory meatloaf has three secret ingredients – Worcestershire sauce, Parmesan cheese, and soy sauce. If you're looking for a crowd pleaser, look no further.

Serves: 6
Prep Time: 25 minutes
Cook Time: 60 minutes

Ingredients:

- Cooking spray
- 2 pounds of ground turkey
- 1 cup of quick-cooking oats
- 1/2 cup of Parmesan cheese
- 1/3 cup of ketchup
- 1/3 cup of chopped yellow onion
- 1/4 cup of chopped parsley
- 1/4 cup of Worcestershire sauce
- 2 tablespoons of soy sauce
- 1 1/2 teaspoons of minced thyme leaves
- 1 teaspoon of minced sage leave
- 1/2 teaspoon of pepper
- 2 minced garlic cloves

Directions:

1. Preheat oven to 400
2. Coat 9x5" loaf pan with cooking spray
3. Mix all ingredients in a large bowl and mix with hands.

4. Pour mixture into the pan
5. Bake until cooked through – about 50-60 minutes

Nutritional Facts Per Serving:
Calories: 613
Total Fat: 23g
Cholesterol: 157mg
Sodium: 1121mg
Carbohydrates: 38g
Protein: 63g
Fiber: 5g

Cauliflower Mashed Potatoes

These cauliflower mashed potatoes are a health spin on an old classic. They work well as a side dish. You won't be able to resist the cheesy goodness.

Serves: 8 (about 1/2 cup each)
Prep Time: 20 minutes
Cook Time: 35 minutes

Ingredients:

- 3 pounds of potatoes
- 1 head of cauliflower
- 3 ounces light cream cheese, softened
- 2 tablespoons butter, softened
- Pinch of salt
- Pinch of pepper
- 1/4 cup of chives

Directions:

1. Peel potatoes and trim cauliflower
2. Soften cream cheese in microwave for 30 seconds
3. Soften butter in microwave for 30 seconds
4. Chop chive
5. Boil water over stovetop in medium size pan. Add potatoes, and cauliflower.
6. Reduce heat to a simmer and let sit until potatoes and cauliflower are tender (about 30 minutes)

7. Drain water and then add butter, light cream cheese, salt and pepper.
8. Use a potato masher to mash mixture.
9. Lastly, stir in chives after chopping chive into small pieces.

Nutritional Facts Per Serving:
Calories: 88
Total Fat: 3g
Cholesterol: 8mg
Sodium: 80mg
Carbohydrates: 14g
Protein: 3.1g
Fiber: 2g

ABOUT THE AUTHOR

Annie DePasquale MD is an actively practicing family physician and mother of two - soon-to-be three! When not caring for her family or patients, she is helping to spread good family medicine practices through her writing and social media pursuits.

Visit her at http://www.FamilyDocAnnie.com

She is also on Facebook and Twitter. #FamilyDocAnnie

If you enjoyed this book, please leave a quick review on Amazon. This would be tremendously appreciated.

OTHER BOOKS

Dr. Annie DePasquale's other published books include:

Delectable Diabetes Desserts: 30 Recipes With 10 Carbs or Less

Cooking With Kids: 30 Healthy Recipes Your Kids Will Love To Make

Gluten Free Desserts: 30 Delicious Recipes

Stress Less: 50 Practical Tips to Decrease Your Daily Stress

Stop Smoking Now

FREE BONUS

As a small token of appreciation for purchasing this book, Dr. Annie would like to offer you a free copy of her next health-related e-book.

You can get your free gift by clicking here:

http://www.FamilyDocAnnie.com/cookbook